THE POWER OF
STRETCHING

THE POWER OF
STRETCHING

SIMPLE PRACTICES TO PROMOTE WELLBEING

BOB DOTO

FAIR WINDS

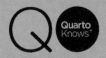

Inspiring | Educating | Creating | Entertaining

Brimming with creative inspiration, how-to projects, and useful information to enrich your everyday life, Quarto Knows is a favorite destination for those pursuing their interests and passions. Visit our site and dig deeper with our books into your area of interest: Quarto Creates, Quarto Cooks, Quarto Homes, Quarto Lives, Quarto Drives, Quarto Explores, Quarto Gifts, or Quarto Kids.

First Published in 2020 by Fair Winds Press,
an imprint of The Quarto Group.
100 Cummings Center, Suite 265-D,
Beverly, MA 01915, USA.
T (978) 282-9590 F (978) 283-2742

Fair Winds Press titles are also available at discount for retail, wholesale, promotional, and bulk purchase. For details, contact the Special Sales Manager by email at specialsales@quarto.com or by mail at The Quarto Group, Attn: Special Sales Manager, 100 Cummings Center, Suite 265-D, Beverly, MA 01915, USA.

24 23 22 21 20 1 2 3 4 5

ISBN: 978-1-59233-936-5

Digital edition published in 2020

QUAR.328316

Conceived, edited, and designed by Quarto Publishing plc.
6 Blundell Street, London N7 9BH

Editor: Claire Waite Brown
Art Director: Gemma Wilson
Designer: Karin Skånberg
Illustrator: Mallory Wood
Publisher: Samantha Warrington

Printed in Singapore

The information in this book is for educational purposes only. It is not intended to replace the advice of a physician or medical practitioner. Please see your health-care provider before beginning any new health program.

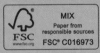

MIX
Paper from responsible sources
FSC® C016973

Contents

Meet Bob

Watch any animal for little more than a few minutes and you will see the ways in which they twist and turn their bodies into what seem to be effortless stretches. Considering how common stretching is within the animal kingdom, it's not hard to understand why one of the questions I hear most often from my massage therapy clients is: "What can I do to stretch out my tight muscles?"

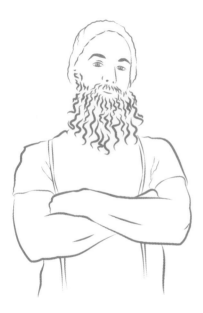

Although I played baseball throughout high school, stretching was something I rarely did with any intention. If I did stretch, I honestly had very little knowledge about what to do or how to do it correctly and effectively. Like many people I knew, I would simply take a limb and extend it in one direction or another until I felt something that *seemed* like a stretch. It wasn't until I began practicing yoga many years ago that I began to understand what this whole stretching thing was about.

With this book I wanted to give you a simple and approachable way to intentionally and effectively stretch every region of your body. There are a number of stretching books on the market, and as a bodyworker I have read most of them. The difference between this book and the others is that this one is for my clients. This is the book I often wish I had so clients could take their treatments home with them and build on what we achieve during bodywork sessions.

However, this is also a book for everyone currently existing in a body. A book I hope will help empower you to take back your ability to increase your sense of wellbeing.

Contraindications

While there are only a few common contraindications for stretching, as with any new physical practice, you may want to consult with your doctor before performing the stretches in this book. And, if you have any pain or known injuries or pathologies that might prevent you from performing these stretches safely, then you definitely want to get the OK from your doctor.

About This Book

Beautiful illustrations, clear text, and an easy-to-access organization within the following pages ensure that you can quickly gain benefits from the power of stretching.

Chapter 1

THE WHYS AND HOWS OF STRETCHING
Pages 10–19

This chapter discusses what intentional stretching is and how it benefits the body and our overall wellbeing. It also features general guidelines on how to perform stretches properly and safely.

Chapter 2

THE STRETCHES
Pages 20–97

Working from the head down, over 60 stretches are detailed in this chapter, with instructions and illustrations to make sure you can replicate and get the most from each exercise.

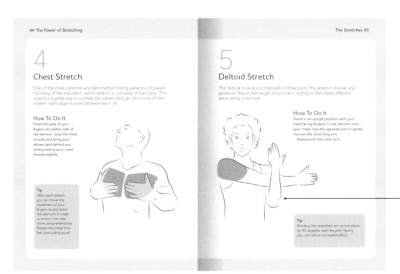

Each stretch is described using an image, written instructions, and extra notes or tips.

Chapter 3

**WHICH STRETCHES
TO USE**
Pages 98–125

The final chapter deals with some of the most common activities modern humans engage in (occupational and sports-related), as well as injuries and repetitive stress conditions, and suggests a number of stretches to perform that can be helpful for each condition or activity. Feel free to do more or less of what's suggested. As there are a number of stretches that affect regions of the body in slightly different ways, you may find that replacing some with others, or adding additional stretches, works for you.

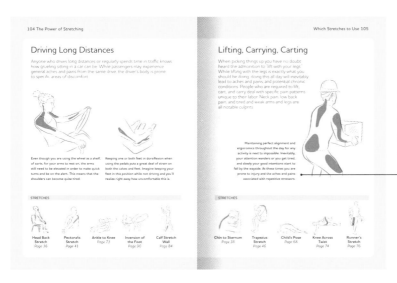

Information is given on how the activity/ injury relates to the body.

CHAPTER 1
THE WHYS AND HOWS OF STRETCHING

In this chapter, you will learn the basics of soft-tissue anatomy and the benefits of stretching. There are also guidelines on how best to perform the stretches, working in conjunction with the breath.

What are Muscles?

The primary functions of muscles are to move our limbs and help us lift heavy objects. However, there are other, in some ways more important, functions associated with healthy muscles.

What Don't They Do?

Muscles help keep all of our internal organs organized and in their place, so that they function properly. Muscles stabilize the body when performing activities. They allow us to breathe, help to circulate the blood, and facilitate digestion. In short, without muscles we would not be able to live.

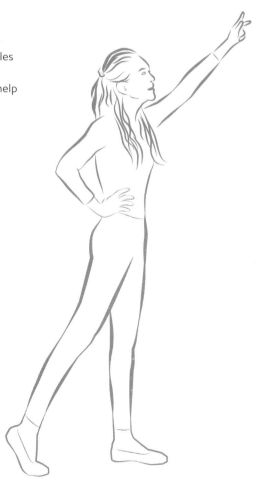

What is a Stretch?

Whether you are an athlete, a truck driver, a nurse, or a cave-dwelling yogi (or an apartment-dwelling yogi), you stretch. When you take a step and press your foot down onto the ground, the plantar fascia on the bottom of the foot stretches. When you stand up from sitting, the movement stretches your hamstrings. Without the ability to stretch muscles you would be virtually immobile, and each one of these "unintentional stretches" has the effect of taking a muscle from a shortened state to a lengthened one.

Intentional Stretching

If you were to exist solely within the limits of these forms of basic movements, your body would, over time, begin to feel very stuck. This is because limited and habitual movement patterns cannot make up for the many ways in which we perpetually hold our bodies in contraction.

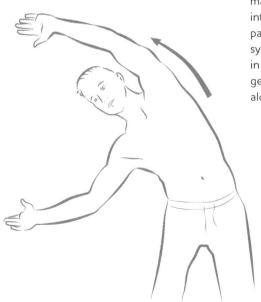

When your muscles stretch from everyday activities, you elongate their fibers—the individual strands that make up the muscle itself. When you intentionally and slowly stretch a muscle past its maximal resting length, with synchronized breathing, as you might in a yoga class, misaligned muscle fibers get the chance to reorganize themselves along the line of the stretch.

The Benefits of Stretching

Creating and maintaining healthy, oxygenated, well-vasculated (blood-enriched) muscle tissue through regular muscle stretching will lead not only to a healthier life, but also a far more enhanced experience of life itself.

Stretching has been shown to be far more than simply a way to feel good. Stretching also:

Increases blood flow to muscles, therefore increasing the rate of rehabilitation after working out or injury.

Relieves stress.

Increases flexibility and range of motion.

Relaxes the nervous system and calms the mind.

Helps prevent injury by conditioning the muscles to be more alert and responsive to stimuli.

Helps increase athletic performance ability.

Soft Tissue

There are three forms of soft tissue that move the body and limbs, stabilize the joints, and help the organs perform their functions.

Muscles

Skeletal muscles attach to the skeletal body. This muscle tissue is considered voluntary, which means that we have control over its use and function.

Smooth muscle fibers line the walls of hollow organs. These fibers are considered involuntary, in that they function without our conscious control.

The cardiac muscle tissue is specific to the walls of the heart. Like smooth muscle, cardiac muscle tissue is involuntary, where the complete set of fibers contracts simultaneously to push blood out from within the heart.

Fascia

Basically speaking, fascia is a tightly woven, fibrous connective tissue that is found throughout the entire body, making its way through the muscle tissue, around individual muscle fibers, and encapsulating groups of muscle bellies. It is often compared to the white fibrous material surrounding and interwoven throughout a peeled orange.

Fascia helps to protect our muscles from each other and other structures in the body, as well as organize and support the structure and performance of the muscles. Over time, fascia and its functions have been the subject of innumerable studies, and, as more is learned, interest in this mysterious tissue continues to increase.

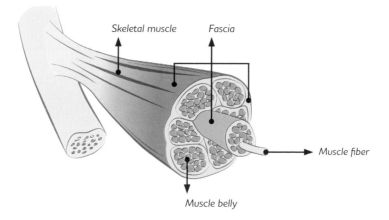

Skeletal muscle Fascia

Muscle fiber

Muscle belly

Stretch the Muscles

Muscles are the most elastic of the soft tissues. Tendons are less so, but still retain some elasticity to accommodate movements in the body, and ligaments have hardly any elasticity at all.

Stretching exercises primarily stretch the muscle bellies. We intentionally do not stretch tendons or ligaments, which can not only cause pain and discomfort but, in the case of ligaments, permanent damage.

Tendons

Tendons are fibrous connective tissue that attach muscles to bones, as well as other soft structures such as the eyeballs. The main function of a tendon is to move the bone or structure. While the muscle belly is what generates the strength needed to move a bone or structure, the tendon, because of its attachment to the structure itself, is what moves it.

Ligaments

You might think of ligaments as taut bandages that connect bone to bone, and in some cases, wrap our many joints. Ligaments are, in a way, what keep our joints stable, making sure each bone or bony protrusion is protected.

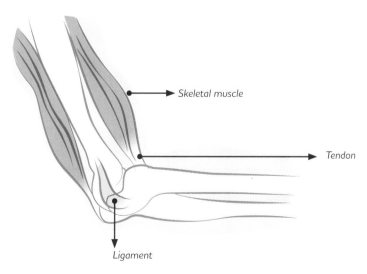

Skeletal muscle

Tendon

Ligament

Stretching Safely

During stretching exercises the muscles should be in the optimal, most supple condition so as to lengthen without injury. Muscle tension is in part directly linked to the state of the nervous system. Think of any time you've been on edge, and you may remember your body tensing up. This sensation is created in part by tension in the muscle tissue. Taking long, deep, intentional breaths, and matching these breaths with movements, helps to relax the muscles and allows for smooth, pain-free stretching.

Stretch with Breath

All body stretches should be done in conjunction with intentional inhales and exhales. In almost all cases, and certainly for the purposes of this particular book, you want to inhale to prepare for the stretch and exhale to perform the stretch. In other words, you exhale to "come into" the stretch.

Length and Frequency

There are a number of opinions on how long to hold a stretch. For this book it is recommended that you hold each stretch for approximately one to two inhales and exhales, and that you repeat each stretch once or twice.

"Listen" to Your Body

Do not overdo it. More does not equal better when it comes to stretching. You are simply looking to feel a shift in the tissues of the area you are stretching. Look for a (sometimes subtle) "opening" sensation in the muscle.

Take a breath in before the stretch.

Breathe out as you move into the stretch.

Hold the stretch for the duration of one to two inhales and exhales.

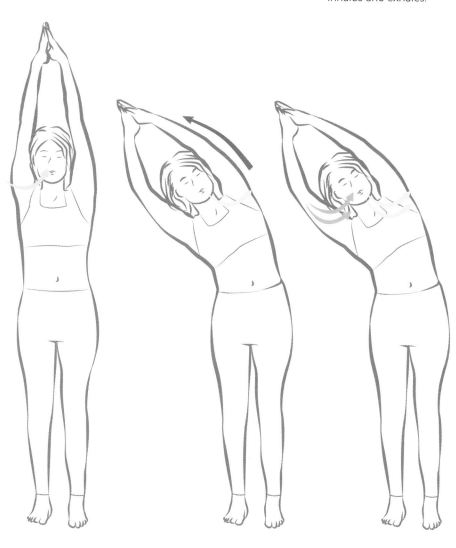

CHAPTER 2
THE STRETCHES

Over 60 stretches are featured in the following chapter, with clear, step-by-step text and illustrations that describe the position and indicate the area of the body being stretched. Tips and safety considerations are provided where necessary.

Stretch Locator

Within this chapter the stretches are grouped according to areas of the body, from the head down to the feet. The graphics on these two pages show the key muscle groups. Some readers may choose systematically to work each group of muscles or to focus on one or two groups, or to look at one muscle within a group.

Back

FACE AND HEAD
pages 24–31

7. Top of Head Squeeze

NECK pages 32–39

3. Chin to Sternum
6. Toward the Armpit

SHOULDERS, CHEST, AND UPPER BACK pages 40–47

6. Trapezius Stretch
7. Thread the Needle

ARMS, HANDS, WRISTS, AND FINGERS pages 48–59

1. Triceps Stretch
3. Full Arm Wall Stretch
4. Forearm Extensor Stretch
6. Wrist Stretch
11. De Quervain's Stretch

ABDOMEN AND LOW BACK pages 60–71

7. Forward Fold
8. Child's Pose
9. Knees to Chest
10. Latissimus Dorsi Stretch
11. Double Knees Across Twist

HIPS AND UPPER LEGS
pages 72–81

1. Ankle to Knee
6. Seated Forward Fold

LOWER LEGS
pages 82–87

1. Calf Stretch Lunge
2. Calf Stretch Wall

ANKLES, FEET, AND TOES pages 88–97

1. Achilles Stretch
4. Plantar Fascia Stretch
6. Toe Extension
7. Toe Spreading
8. Spreading Top and Bottom of Foot
9. Tennis Ball Stretch

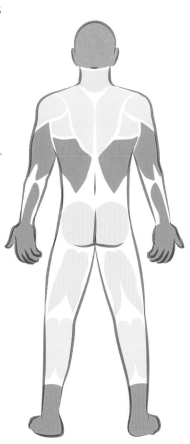

Front

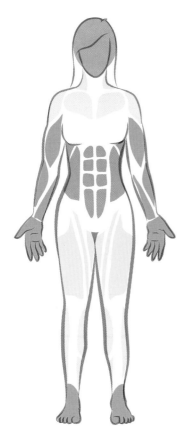

STRETCHES FOR THE
FACE AND HEAD

1

Eye Stretches

Like all muscles in the body, the small muscles of the eyes can become tired from overuse. Eye stretches can offer relief, and can have a very soothing effect on tension-derived headaches.

How To Do It

Begin by looking straight ahead. Then look up, down, left, and right in that order. Hold each stationary position for the duration of a breath—for example: inhale and look up; exhale and look down.

Next, make half-circle motions, arcing toward the forehead first, followed by half circles in the direction of the feet. Alternate the breaths for the half circles as you go back and forth, so that you inhale in one direction and exhale on the way back.

Further Considerations

Do not overexert or hold these positions for too long—repeating just once or twice should be sufficient.

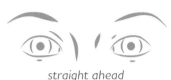

straight ahead

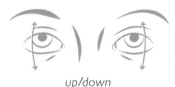

up/down

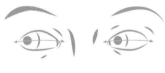

left/right

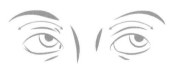

half circles up

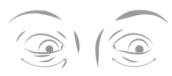

half circles down

2

Looking Into the Distance

Looking at screens for many hours can be incredibly stressful on the eyes. By holding focus on a screen our eye muscles tire, which can lead to headaches and wooziness. If you find yourself looking at screens all day, make time to relieve the strain on your eyes by looking off into the distance.

How To Do It

Stand or sit looking out of a window. Focus your eyes on a point in the distance. The objective is to engage the muscles that focus the eyes.

Further Considerations

Sometimes focusing on a specific point can feel strenuous. If this is the case, looking at a general landscape far away can be enough to engage the muscles in the eyes, and will suffice.

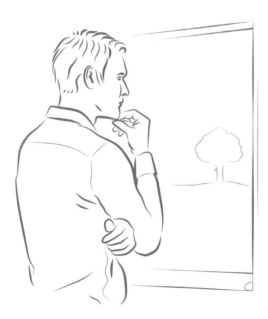

Tip
If you are not by a window, then find a point in the room that is in the distance.

3

Ear Stretches

Because of their proximity to the head and scalp, stretching the ears can have a very relieving effect on headaches and general tenderness around the eyes, head, and face.

How To Do It

Make a hook shape with your index finger and extend your thumb out slightly. Press the hooked finger flat against the opening of the ear, as if you were trying to close or cover it. With the thumb behind the ear, press the index finger and thumb together and make gentle stretches forward toward the face, backward, up, and down.

Further Considerations

Do not stretch the ears too hard. You should not hear any popping or feel any discomfort. A little goes a long way when it comes to stretching the ears.

Tip
You don't want to pinch or pull on the ears, so avoid using the tips of your fingers and thumbs.

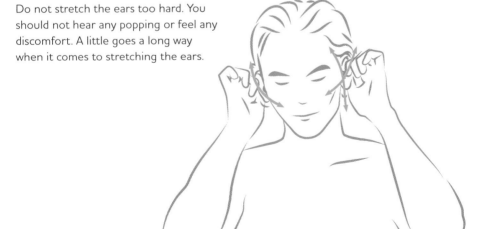

4

Around the Eyes

The face is one of the main areas of the body where tension is stored. Take a few moments every day to perform these stretches so the small but powerful muscles around the eyes get some relief.

How To Do It

Press the pads of the fingers on your temples and gently pull the skin back toward the hairline.

Next, with your eyes closed, press the pads of the fingers just beneath the eyebrows and gently press them toward the forehead.

Finally, press the pads of the fingers into the skin just below the cheekbones. Keeping your head in a neutral position, look up toward the forehead while you pull down on the skin beneath the fingers.

Tip
Making small circles with your fingers as you apply pressure can be very soothing.

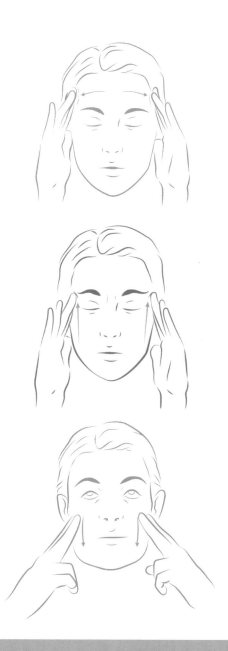

5

Open Mouth Stretch

At some point throughout the day, most people will unintentionally contract various muscle groups (glutes, fists, shoulders, etc.). For many people, clenching the muscles around the jaw is the main culprit. Find time each day to open your mouth wide, even if you need to pretend you're yawning!

How To Do It

Massage the muscles around the jaw with the pads of your fingers to warm them up. Open the mouth wide.

Further Considerations

If you have TMJD or "clicking" of the jaw when opening the mouth, do not open the mouth as wide as possible. Instead, follow the Alternative exercise.

Alternative

If you are unable to open the mouth fully, partially open it to your level of comfort. Take hold of the inside of the mouth with the ring and index finger while pressing into each with the thumb on the outside of the mouth. From there, make gentle stretches up and down.

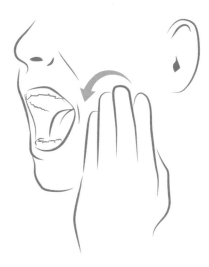

6

Tongue Out

Every culture has its own acceptable forms of bodily expressions. In the West, sticking out one's tongue is not one of them. Nevertheless, it's important to give our tongues, one of the strongest and most overused muscles, a good stretch whenever we can.

How To Do It

Massage the muscles around the jaw with the pads of the fingers to warm them up.

Open the mouth wide and stick out your tongue as far as you can.

Further Considerations

The tongue is considered the most flexible muscle in the body. As such, adapting this stretch by holding the tongue in different positions (up, down, left, right) can be very rewarding.

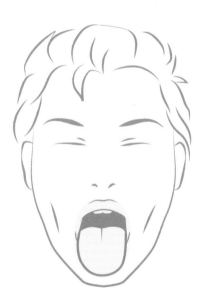

Tip

Making a strong exhale when you stick out your tongue will enhance the stretch. In yoga, this is known as Lion's Breath.

7

Top of Head Squeeze

There are many stretches and massage techniques we can do to relieve the pain of a headache. Squeezing the top of the head in order to relax the thin muscles covering the skull is essential.

How To Do It

Interlace the fingers above your head while pressing the root of your palm into the area, about 2 inches (5 cm) above the ears. Squeeze the hands together, making your way up toward the crown of the head.

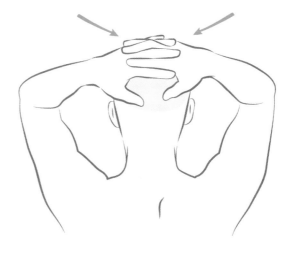

Further Considerations

This stretch, along with eye stretches, can have a very soothing effect on tension-derived headaches.

Tip
Pressing directly into the head puts pressure on the skull, which you want to avoid, so try to engage the skin and thin muscle tissue just beneath the skin by squeezing in a slightly upward direction.

STRETCHES FOR THE
NECK

1

Turning the Head

Decreased range of motion when turning the head is one of the most common neck pathologies. Done with intention, this stretch can yield great benefits.

How To Do It

Looking forward, bring your head into a comfortable neutral position. On an exhale, turn the head to one side. On the inhale, bring the head back to the center.

Repeat the step to turn the head in the opposite direction.

Further Considerations

As with all stretches, do not rush. Taking your time is especially important when stretching the neck.

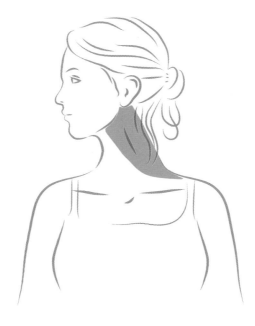

2

Traction Below the Collarbone

Sometimes just a simple procedural addition to a stretch can make all the difference. For this neck stretch, pay close attention to the placement of the fingers.

How To Do It

Press the pads of your fingers just below the collarbone while extending the head up and back.

Repeat on the other side.

Further Considerations

As with all the stretches, a little bit can go a long way. Do not overdo it!

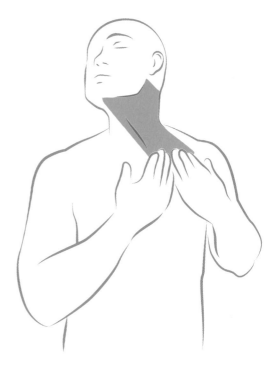

Tip
To increase the depth of the stretch, pull down slightly with the fingers.

3

Chin to Sternum

The advent of the smartphone means that the head-forward posture has practically become an epidemic, so you might be surprised by how good it feels to bring the chin to the sternum to stretch the back of the neck.

How To Do It

Tilt your head down so that your chin is pressing into or close to the sternum.

Place your dominant hand on top of your head with the fingers facing the back. Lightly traction the head forward to increase the stretch.

Repeat on the other side.

Further Considerations

You should feel a comfortable stretch to the back of the neck. If you feel any discomfort on the throat, you're pulling too hard, so relax the pressure.

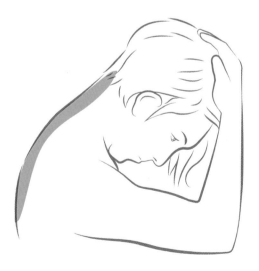

Tip
Place the chin into the sternum first, before applying traction with the hand on the head.

4

Head Back Stretch

This stretch is particularly useful for people who find themselves looking at their phones or other electronic devices for many hours a day. In other words, all of us!

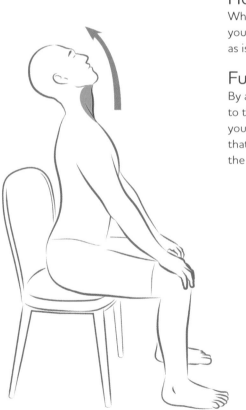

How To Do It

While sitting down or standing, and with your spine long, tilt your head back as far as is comfortable.

Further Considerations

By adding a slightly stronger contraction to the muscles on the back of your neck, you can potentially relieve stress or tension that might be present around the base of the skull.

Tip
To increase the intensity of the stretch, press your fingers just below the collarbone as you tilt your head back.

5

Lateral Neck Stretch

The neck is comprised of many muscles, tendons, and ligaments. Perform this stretch slowly, making sure not to pull or tug on the head.

How To Do It

Hold the seat of the chair with one hand—the same hand as the stretch. Place the other hand on top of the head and gently traction it in the opposite direction.

Repeat on the other side.

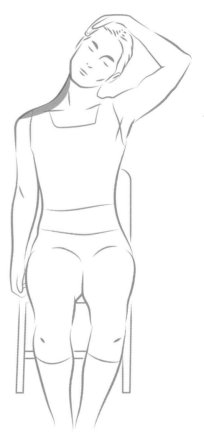

Tip

Holding onto the chair prevents the shoulder rising during the stretch, which would make it less effective.

6

Toward the Armpit

While this stretch can be done sitting or standing, the sitting position allows you to maintain a depressed shoulder while holding onto the chair.

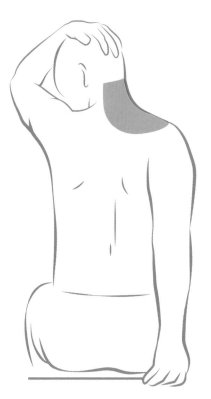

How To Do It

Sit upright in a chair, looking forward, with a straight spine. Hold the seat of the chair with one hand—the same hand as the stretch. Tilt the head forward and down at an angle, as if you are looking at your opposite armpit.

Place the other hand on top of the head and gently traction the head down at an angle toward the armpit.

Repeat on the other side.

Tip
Holding onto the chair prevents the shoulder rising during the stretch, which would make it less effective.

7

Back and Away

Be mindful that you do not overdo this stretch in an effort to "feel it more." Necks can be sensitive, and even if you are not feeling an intense stretch, it does not mean the muscles aren't being positively affected.

How To Do It

Sit upright in a chair with your head facing forward. Turn the head to one side and look up and back behind you.

Further Considerations

If you feel any strain in the neck, slowly come out of the stretch and rest.

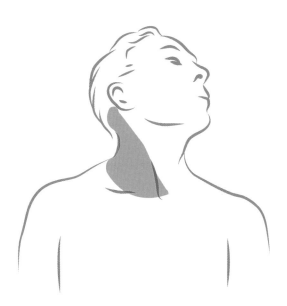

Tip

A simple trick to increase the effect of the stretch is to stretch your mouth in the direction you are turning. This will engage muscles in the face and superficial muscles of the neck.

STRETCHES FOR THE SHOULDERS, CHEST, AND UPPER BACK

1

Pectoralis Stretch

Many people perform this stretch instinctually, because it's easy to do and just feels really great!

How To Do It

Standing up, look straight ahead. Interlace your fingers behind your back and roll the shoulders back as far as is comfortable.

Alternatives

If you are able, turn the palms away from you to increase this stretch.

Another alternative is to leave the hands in the original neutral position and lift the arms slightly.

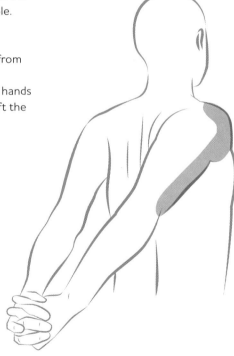

Tip
You can increase the effectiveness of this common stretch with deep inhales and exhales.

2

Doorway Pectoralis Stretch

Using objects and structures in your environment can be a great way to increase the effects of a stretch. Don't be afraid to be "that person" at the party using a doorway to relieve those overworked pecs!

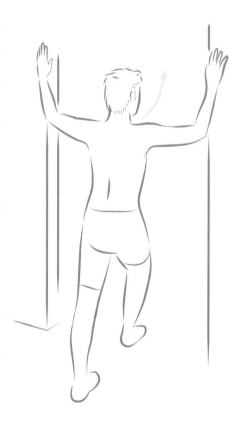

How To Do It

Stand in a doorway. Spread your arms wide in a "cactus" shape, placing your forearms on the inside of the door frame. Step one foot forward in a gentle lunge and lean into the doorway.

Further Considerations

Don't lean into the doorway without stepping one foot forward. Doing so causes the pecs to engage to prevent you from falling, which is the opposite of what you want to happen.

Tips

You can also do this stretch one arm at a time.

If performing this stretch with both arms simultaneously, changing the forward foot can help to increase the stretch.

3

Bolster Pectoralis Stretch

Allowing muscles to stretch without assistance is called passive stretching. Forms of passive stretching, like allowing the pecs to stretch on their own while resting on a bolster, can often be done for slightly longer periods of time than active stretches.

How To Do It

Lay on the floor with a bolster propped up down the center of your back, from the sacrum to the back of the head. With your arms out to the side in a "T" shape, turn the palms to face up.

Alternatives

If you prefer, you can position the arms at your sides, or place them in a "cactus" position, bent at the elbows.

Tip

If you don't own a bolster, you can make one out of rolled-up towels or blankets. Just be sure that whatever you use is firm enough to keep your back slightly arched.

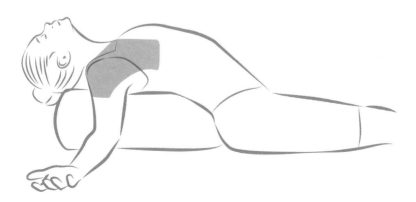

4

Chest Stretch

One of the most common and detrimental holding patterns is forward rounding of the shoulders, which leads to a concavity of the chest. This stretch is a great way to combat the pattern and get into some of the smaller intercostal muscles between each rib.

How To Do It

Press the pads of your fingers into either side of the sternum. Grip the chest muscles and bring your elbows back behind you while pressing your chest forward slightly.

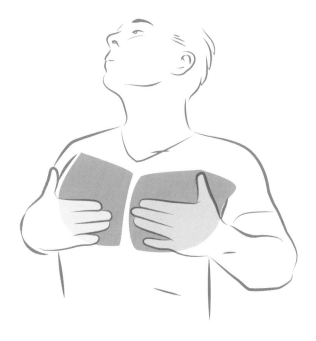

Tip
After each stretch you can move the placement of your fingers up and down the sternum in order to stretch the area more comprehensively. Repeat any areas that feel particularly good!

5

Deltoid Stretch

The deltoid muscle is comprised of three parts: the anterior, medial, and posterior. Adjust the height of your arm slightly to feel these different areas being stretched.

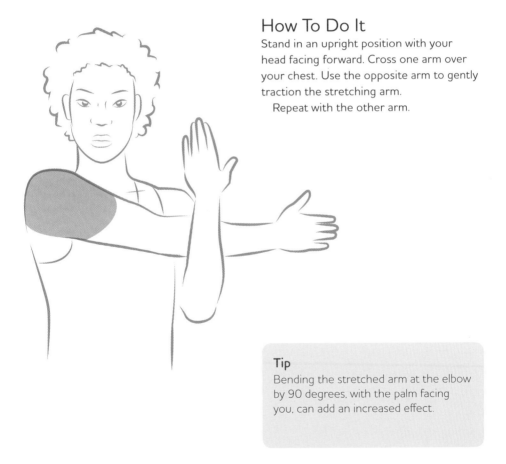

How To Do It

Stand in an upright position with your head facing forward. Cross one arm over your chest. Use the opposite arm to gently traction the stretching arm.

Repeat with the other arm.

Tip
Bending the stretched arm at the elbow by 90 degrees, with the palm facing you, can add an increased effect.

6

Trapezius Stretch

The trapezius muscle covers a large portion of the back, yet it is rarely intentionally stretched. Once you find the sweet spot with this stretch, you may find yourself doing it every day!

How To Do It

Sit in a chair. Lean forward slightly and grab the outside of each opposite thigh with your hands. Slowly start to lean back while rounding the spine, and at the same time resist this movement with the hands grabbing the thighs.

Further Considerations

This can sometimes be a difficult stretch for people to feel. You may need to increase the rounding of the back and the resistance from the hands in order to properly feel this stretch.

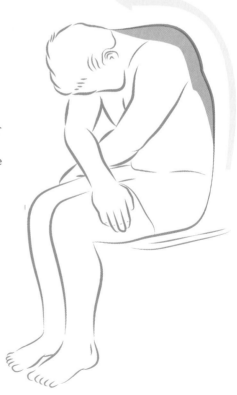

7

Thread the Needle

Many people find this stretch to be one of the most relieving for general shoulder tightness and tension. Perhaps that's why so many mainstream yoga classes make time to play with this pose.

How To Do It

Starting in an all-fours position, take one arm and thread it behind the other until the outside of your shoulder is resting on the floor.

Further Considerations

You may need to sink down toward your heels if you are finding it difficult to rest your shoulder on the floor.

Tip

To experience the fullest expression of this stretch, be sure to walk the non-stretched arm overhead, while placing the side of your head on the floor. At the same time bring your gaze toward the ceiling.

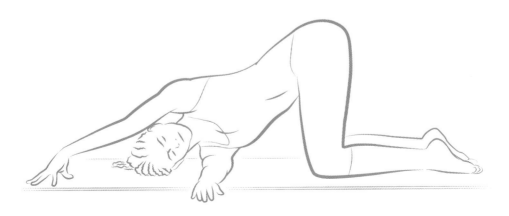

STRETCHES FOR THE
ARMS, HANDS, WRISTS, AND FINGERS

1

Triceps Stretch

Perhaps it's because of their placement on the back of the arm (an area of the body we don't regularly see in the mirror), but these primary arm extensor muscles are often overlooked when it comes to stretching.

How To Do It

Stretch one arm up alongside your head. Bend this arm at the elbow so your fingers are facing down your back with the palm facing the back. With the opposite hand, gently press the elbow down and slightly back to feel the stretch.

Repeat with the other arm.

Further Considerations

Do not press too hard on the elbow. Adding simple and gentle pressure should be enough to engage the stretch. For some people no pressure at all will be needed.

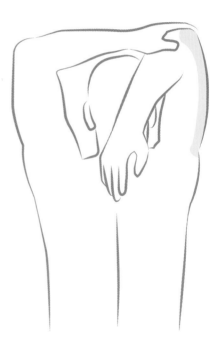

Tip

If you are flexible enough, rather than pressing the elbow from above, you can reach the opposite hand up around the back and clasp both hands. Alternatively, you can use a strap or towel if your hands will not reach.

2

Biceps Wall Stretch

There are many ways to stretch the biceps. However, this stretch is one of the most comprehensive, where the benefits are easiest to experience.

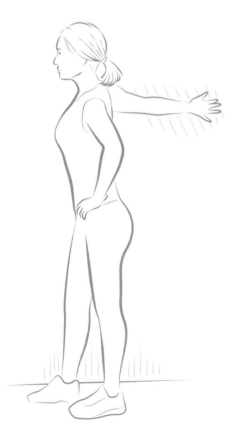

How To Do It

Stand alongside a wall with one arm stretched back behind you, and your palm flat on the wall. Step one foot forward while leaning slightly in the direction of the foot. Repeat on the other side.

Further Considerations

If you feel any pains in your shoulder while performing this stretch, then put more space between you and the wall to decrease the intensity.

Tip

Try alternating the forward-stepping foot, to feel which better facilitates the stretch.

3

Full Arm Wall Stretch

The fascial lines of the arm extend from the shoulder down to the fingers. Performing this stretch will have a lengthening effect on this entire line of connective tissue.

How To Do It

Stand alongside a wall with one arm outstretched and your palm against the wall with your fingers facing back. Slowly turn away from the wall until you feel a stretch along the entire arm and hand. Repeat on the other side.

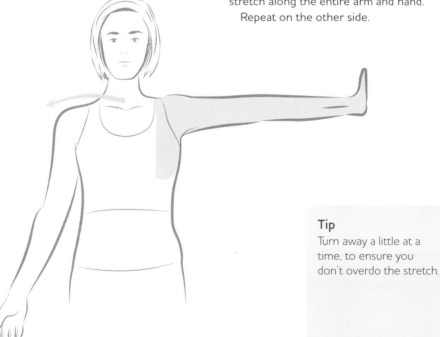

Tip

Turn away a little at a time, to ensure you don't overdo the stretch.

4

Forearm Extensor Stretch

With today's reliance on typing and texting, the forearms have become some of the most overused, yet under-cared-for, muscles in the body. You can perform this stretch whenever the need arises.

How To Do It

Outstretch one arm with the palm facing down. Clasp the top of the outstretched hand with the opposite hand and traction the fingers down until you feel the muscles of the forearm stretching.

Repeat with the other arm.

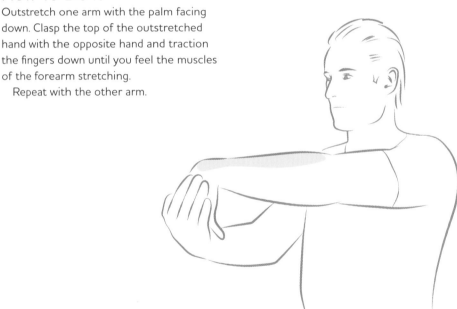

Tip

To increase the intensity of the stretch, curl the fingers of the outstretched hand into a fist.

5

Forearm Flexor Stretch

Our modern-day reliance on typing and texting means that the forearms are often overused. Perform this stretch whenever the need arises.

How To Do It

Extend one arm out in front of you with the palm facing up. With the opposite hand, press the outstretched fingers down toward the floor.

Repeat with the other arm.

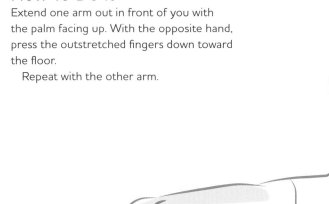

Tip

To increase the stretch, begin to lower the arm.

6

Wrist Stretch

Wrists are more than just hinges from which the hand flops up and down. Add a gentle twist to stretch the wrist in order to get the most out of your wrist's flexibility.

How To Do It

Bend your elbow so that your palm is facing you at the level of your face. Wrap your opposite hand around the back of the hand, placing your thumb behind the base of the pinky and allowing the fingers to grab the wrist lightly on the side of the thumb.

Gently turn the hand, using the fingers to grip the far side of the wrist and the thumb to press the pinky finger toward you.

Further Considerations

Be careful not to overdo this stretch. Twisting of any kind should be done with care and attention to any discomfort.

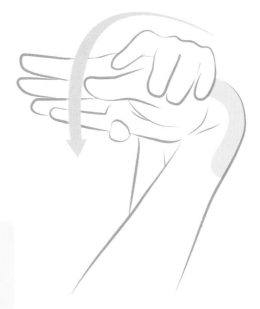

Tip
The fingers of the hand and wrist being stretched should be spread and not locked down together.

7

Palms Out Stretch

This is one of the most intuitive stretches that people do, and can be done as often as needed.

How To Do It

Interlace your fingers close to, and at the level of, the chest.

On an exhale, press the palms away from you until your arms become straight.

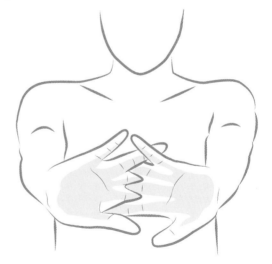

Tips

To increase the effect, slightly round your upper back to feel the stretch through the back of the shoulders.

You can also try doing this with the hands stretched overhead.

Tented Fingers

You might be surprised by how relieving this stretch is after a long day at the office, playing sports, or even just sitting around on a hot and humid day when the hands tend to swell.

How To Do It

Line up the pads of each finger and thumb while holding the hands at the level of the chest.

Press the palms of your hands toward one another until the fingers and thumbs are spread out in a stretched position.

Further Considerations

While the hands are typically very mobile, be sure not to overstretch the fingers and thumbs by pressing the palms too strongly toward one another. Press only to the point where you feel the stretch engaging.

Tip

To achieve a more comprehensive stretch, try to specifically stretch the thumbs away from the rest of the fingers, while at the same time spreading the fingers away from each other.

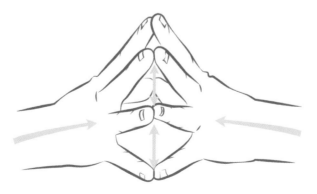

9

Thumb Stretch Down

Surprising to many people, but one of the most tender areas of our muscle tissue can be found around the thumbs. Use this stretch to help relieve some of the inevitable tension that comes with our increased dependency on smartphones and electronic devices.

How To Do It
With a bent elbow, hold your hand out in front of you with your fingers pointing back at you. Use the opposite thumb to stretch the thumb down and away from you.

Further Considerations
The thumbs are comprised of many muscles, tendons, and ligaments. Perform the stretch slowly, making sure not to pull too hard.

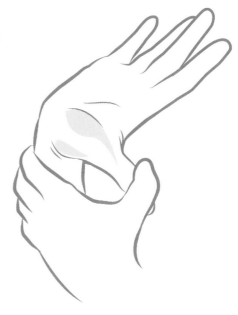

Tip
Use the fingers of the hand performing the stretch to hold onto the opposite arm, which will help give leverage to the stretch.

10

Finkelstein Stretch

This and any other thumb and finger stretch can be used as part of a comprehensive stretch regimen for the hands and palms.

How To Do It

With a bent elbow, hold your hand out in front of you with the palm facing up. Reach under the forearm with your opposite hand and hold the thumb of the outstretched hand. Gently stretch the thumb down and back toward the wrist.

Further Considerations

The thumbs are comprised of many muscles, tendons, and ligaments. Perform the stretch slowly, making sure you don't pull too hard.

Be mindful not to overdo this stretch.

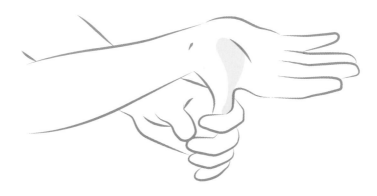

11

De Quervain's Stretch

This seemingly simple stretch lengthens the tendons of the wrist just behind the thumb, and can feel very tender. It is named after the muscle test that assesses whether these tendons are irritated.

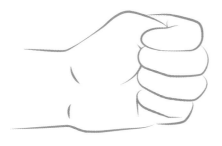

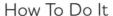

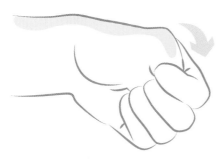

How To Do It

Hold your hand out in front of you with the palm facing in and the thumb on top. Wrap the fingers around the thumb. Bend the wrist down toward the floor.

Repeat with the other hand.

Tip

Because of the direction in which your hand is facing, the wrist will only bend slightly, much less than if your palm was facing down.

STRETCHES FOR THE
ABDOMEN AND LOW BACK

1

Ab Stretch

Stretching the abdomen is particularly helpful, and necessary, if you have been performing abdominal exercise or workouts. Ironically, stretching the abdomen is also helpful if you have not been working out your abdominal muscles, since they are often shortened due to slouching in a chair.

How To Do It

Standing with your feet hip-width apart, roll your shoulders back while bringing your hands down to your buttocks.

Tilt your head back slightly, lift your belly out of the pelvis, and gently lean back, sliding your hands down toward the back of your legs.

Further Considerations

Lifting the belly out of the pelvis is very important to keep the low back from compressing. This lift will also help to increase the effectiveness of the stretch.

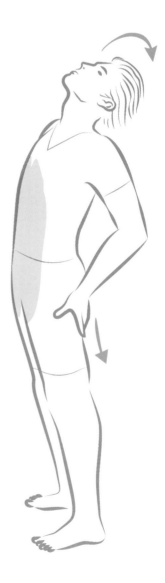

2

Ab Twist

This ab stretch is helpful after a workout, or for those who spend a lot of time seated.

How To Do It

With your arms stretched overhead, interlace the fingers with the palms facing upward, then place the palms on the back of the head. Slowly turn to one side on an exhale.

Repeat to the opposite side.

Alternative

If it is comfortable to do so, you can slightly arch your back in order to increase the effects on the abdomen. Only do this after you have turned to one side: do not arch while you are twisting.

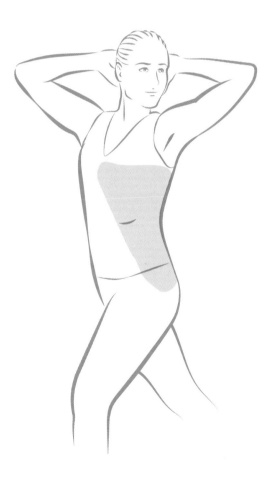

3

Stability Ball Stretch

Using a stability ball to stretch the abdomen while extending the arms up overhead can be very helpful in understanding the relationship between the arms, the abdomen, and the sides of the body. A lengthened core can really help to give freedom to the movement of your arms.

How To Do It

Sit on the stability ball with your feet hip-width apart. Walk your feet out until you are laying on the ball.

Once you are stable, take your arms over your head and press into your feet as you arch your back over the ball.

Further Considerations

Only go as far back as is comfortable, and to the point where you can feel the abdominal muscles stretching.

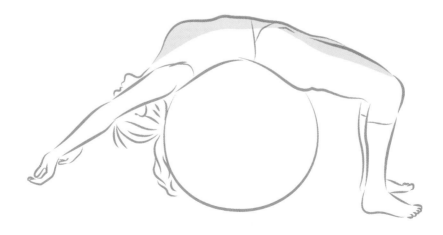

4

Cobra Stretch

A typical yoga class will often incorporate a number of "chest openers," including variations of the cobra stretch.

How To Do It

Lay with your belly on the floor. Place your palms under your shoulders with your elbows bent alongside you. On an inhale, press your palms into the floor as you lift your chest and belly away from the floor.

Alternative

To modify this pose, keep your forearms on the floor and only come up to where is comfortable.

Further Considerations

To engage the abdominal muscles, you only need to press up as much as is comfortable.

Tip
Avoid splaying your elbows out to the sides, but rather keep them in tight.

5

Side Stretch

Just because many of us used to do this stretch in gym class as children does not make it a has-been of the stretching world. Its effects are as significant today as they have always been.

How To Do It

Standing with your feet apart, raise one arm up alongside your ear with the palm facing your head. On an exhale, reach the hand up and over your head as you lean to one side.

Repeat on the other side.

Further Considerations

Using a mirror can be helpful when attempting to reach out of the abdomen, rather than just leaning to one side: you can see that your abdomen is lengthening.

Tip

Bring your awareness to your belly as you do this stretch, and, rather than simply leaning to one side, try to reach up and out of the abdomen.

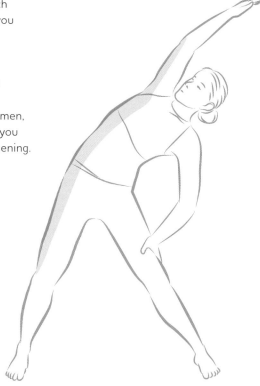

6

Side Stretch with Twist

This stretch is very similar to the previous stretch (see page 65) with only a few minor, but significant, additions to help you access the quadratus lumborum muscle (the QL), which is often one of the most aggravated of all the muscles in the low back.

How To Do It

Standing with your feet apart, raise one arm up alongside your ear with the palm facing your head. On an exhale, reach your hand up and over your head as you lean to one side.

Once in your end position, slightly turn the body and lean forward. You will only need to lean about an inch or so to engage the small stabilizer muscles of the low back.

Repeat on the other side.

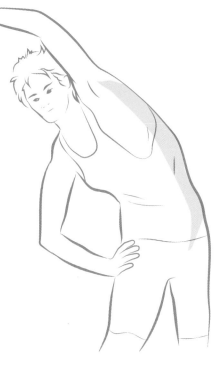

Further Considerations

It may take some finessing of the stretch to truly find the stabilizing muscles of the low back. Gently refine the stretch at slightly different angles until you feel those muscles lengthening.

Tip

Bring your awareness to your belly as you do this stretch, and, rather than simply leaning to one side, try to reach up and out of the abdomen.

7

Forward Fold

Despite being one of the simplest stretches to instruct people to do, folding forward over the legs can be a challenge for many people.

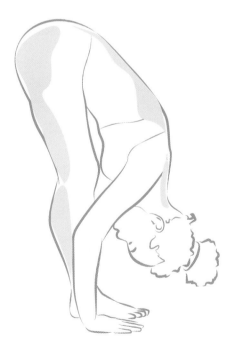

How To Do It

Stand with your feet hip-width apart with your hands on your waist. Bring a slight bend to your knees and slowly fold forward over your legs.

Alternatives

Once folded, you can either grab opposite elbows over your head with your hands, or, if it is comfortable to do so, place your palms on the floor.

Further Considerations

Depending on the length of your hamstrings and the flexibility in your low back, you may need to modify this stretch by resting your hands or arms on the back of a chair or table. By doing so, you should avoid overlengthening these otherwise short muscles.

8

Child's Pose

Anyone who's ever taken a difficult yoga class will be familiar with this often requested "rest" position.

How To Do It

Sit on your heels and slowly bring your belly to your thighs. Walk your hands out in front of you and place them on the floor with your fingers stretched wide.

Alternative

With your arms outstretched you can walk your hands to the left and the right to isolate and increase the stretch on each side of the body.

Further Considerations

If you are unable to sit on your heels comfortably, place a bolster or a rolled-up blanket on your heels to decrease the distance between them and your butt.

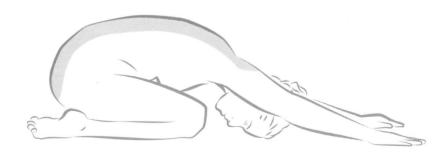

9

Knees to Chest

Because of the position of the knees against the chest, this stretch is in effect very similar to the Child's Pose (see opposite). You may substitute one for the other if either is uncomfortable for you.

How To Do It

Lay on your back and bring one or both knees to your chest. Wrap your arms around the knees and hug them close to the chest.

Tip

Adding space between the knees so that they point out toward your shoulders may help to bring a bit of mobility to the hips.

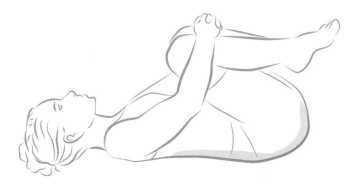

10

Latissimus Dorsi Stretch

The latissimus dorsi muscles, or "lats," are strong muscles that cover much of the low back, but attach just around the armpits. Stretching these muscles is particularly important for people active in swimming, throwing, and climbing.

How To Do It

Stand tall and bring your arms up and slightly behind the ears. Cross one wrist over the other, and stretch upward.

Repeat by alternating the wrist in front.

Further Considerations

By gently pressing the area being stretched out to the side, you can experience the benefits of this stretch more fully.

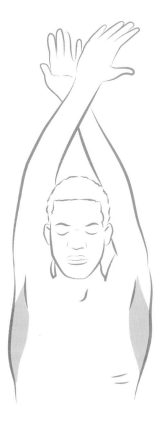

Tip

Be sure to have your head and gaze tipped down toward the floor, to make room for the arms to stretch overhead.

11
Double Knees Across Twist

Despite the fact that this is a huge stretch for the low back and hips, many people find the position restful once they have settled into place. Don't fall asleep!

How To Do It
Lay on your back with your arms outstretched to form a "T" shape. Bring both knees into your chest. Bring one hip slightly off-center to one side, then slowly place your knees on the floor to the opposite side.

Repeat on the other side.

Further Considerations
Do not overdo this stretch. Only bring the knees over as far as is comfortable while still keeping your shoulder on the floor. You may end up not going as far as you might expect, and that is fine.

Tip
Try to keep both shoulders on the floor. If they are rising up, reduce the depth of the stretch by raising the knees.

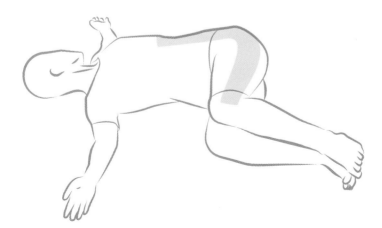

STRETCHES FOR THE
HIPS AND UPPER LEGS

1

Ankle to Knee

This stretch works specifically on your piriformis muscle, which is often aggravated from sitting all day. Because the sciatic nerve runs underneath this muscle, tension in the piriformis can lead to sciatica-like symptoms, such as numbness and achiness down the leg.

How To Do It

While laying on your back, bend one knee so that your foot rests flat on the floor. Place the ankle of the opposite leg on the thigh, just above the knee.

Reach your arms around the bent leg, clasping your hands behind the thigh. Gently bring the leg toward the chest.

Repeat on the other leg.

Alternative

For a slightly less intense version of this stretch, do not bring the leg toward your chest, but rather leave it so that the foot remains resting on the floor.

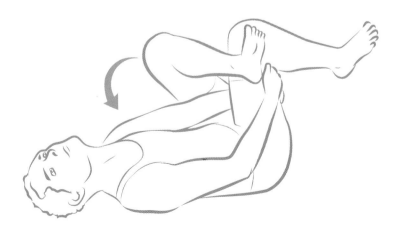

2

Knee Across Twist

This stretch is known for its "Ooh yeah" quality, because it gets into areas of both the low back and hips, which are often in need of relief.

How To Do It

While laying on your back, hug one knee to your chest. On an exhale, slowly bring your knee to the opposite side of your body, using your opposite hand to guide the knee.

Extend the unused arm out to the side and try to keep the shoulder on the floor.

Repeat on the other side.

Further Considerations

Do not overdo this stretch. Only bring the knee over as far as is comfortable while still keeping your shoulder on the floor. You may end up not going as far as you might expect, and that is fine.

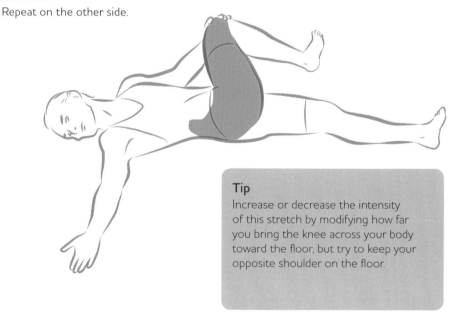

Tip
Increase or decrease the intensity of this stretch by modifying how far you bring the knee across your body toward the floor, but try to keep your opposite shoulder on the floor.

3
Outside Hip Stretch

This stretch engages both the glutes on the back and side of the hip, as well as muscles that cross the front.

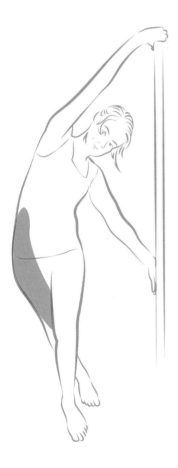

How To Do It

Stand with your hand holding the inside of a door frame. Bring your feet close together and lean into your hip away from the door.

Repeat on the other side.

Tip
You may need to adjust the placement of the outside foot in order to better access this stretch.

4

Runner's Stretch

The most prominent quadricep muscle, rectus femoris, which runs up the center of the upper leg, crosses both the hip and the knee. Sitting all day can leave this muscle feeling tight, especially when going from a sitting to standing position. So, although called a runner's stretch, this stretch is also very important for office workers.

How To Do It

Bend one leg at the knee. Reach around to grab the top of the foot and bring the foot toward your glutes.

   Repeat on the other side.

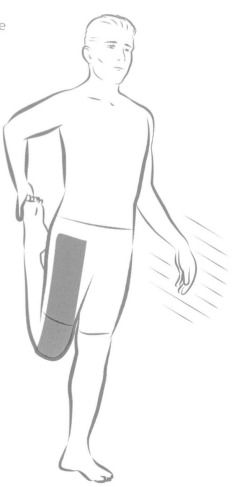

Tips

Stand alongside a wall, using your hand against it to maintain balance.

Increase or decrease the intensity of this stretch by modifying how far you bring the foot toward your glutes.

5

Supta Vajrasana

This stretch is a common yoga posture. It can be very deep and should always be performed in small increments. As you will feel, a little goes a long way with this stretch.

How To Do It

Sit on your heels with your knees roughly hip-width apart. Bring your hands behind you on the floor with your fingers facing forward. Slowly lower yourself down in between your hands.

Tip
Increase or decrease the intensity of this stretch by modifying how far you bring your upper body down toward the floor. The fullest expression of this stretch is to have your back lying flat on the floor behind you, with your hands and arms extended overhead.

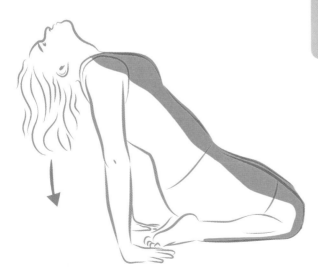

6

Seated Forward Fold

This yoga posture is known as Paschimottanasana, and is one of the most common poses you may encounter in a yoga class. Usually performed with legs resting flat on the floor, this posture is a great lengthener of the entire line of tissue that runs from the back of the legs all the way to the head.

How To Do It

Sit on the floor with your legs together and extended out in front of you. On an inhale, lift your arms up overhead, then on an exhale lengthen through the spine, slowly bringing the arms down and resting the hands as far down the legs as is comfortable.

Alternative

If you find that this stretch is too intense on the back of the legs, sit on a chair or bench and perform the stretch in the same way.

Tip

Make sure that when folding forward you bring your belly toward your thighs and also keep your head in line with your spine, rather than simply rounding your back and dropping the head down.

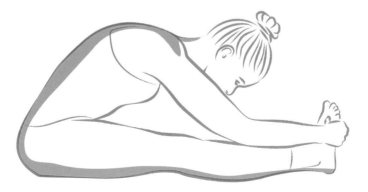

7

Adductors Stretch

Many of us, as children, were taught to do this "butterfly stretch" by vigorously flapping our knees up and down. Avoid doing that at all costs! As with all the stretches in this book, use your breath to slowly engage the stretch for maximum relief.

How To Do It
Sit on the floor with your knees out to the sides and the soles of your feet together. Take hold of your feet with your thumbs wrapped around the soles. Gently lean forward while attempting to keep your knees from lifting.

Further Considerations
Pay close attention to any discomfort or strain in the knees when performing this stretch.

Tip
To increase the lengthening effects of this stretch, walk your hands out in front of you, bringing your belly closer to your feet.

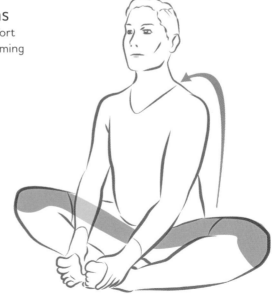

8

Seated Wide Leg

This is a great stretch for so many areas of the lower body and back, and is particularly helpful if you've been sitting all day.

How To Do It

Sit on the floor with your legs spread wide and toes facing up. Bring the hands either to the legs or walk them out in front as you slowly fold forward, making sure to lengthen through the spine, bringing your belly down first.

Tip

To increase the stretch on the back of the legs, try to keep your toes up and your feet straight (not splayed out to the sides). This will lengthen the muscles of the back of the lower leg, so do so gently.

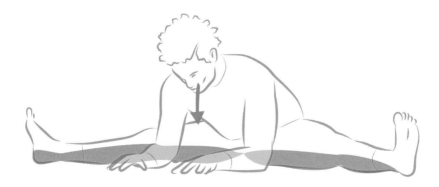

9

Adductors Side Lunge

Your groin muscles—the adductors—are some of the strongest in the body. Consequently, they can get rather stiff.

How To Do It

Standing with your feet wide apart, turn one foot out to the side while bending the opposite knee. Lean toward the bent knee until you feel the stretch in the opposite lengthened leg.

Repeat on the other leg.

Further Considerations

Take care when lunging in this posture and only go as far as is comfortable.

Tip
By rooting down the outside edge of the foot of the long leg you can also partially stretch the outside of that leg.

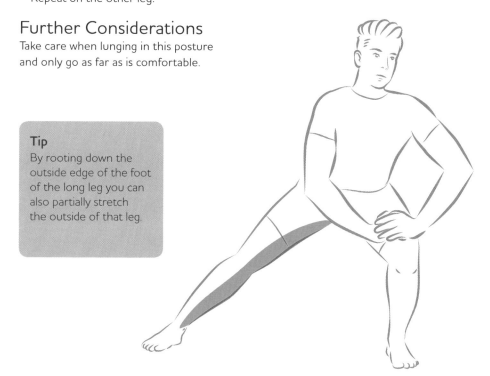

STRETCHES FOR THE
LOWER LEGS

1

Calf Stretch Lunge

This stretch can be used with foot stretches (see pages 90–97) in order to achieve a comprehensive stretch in the entire region.

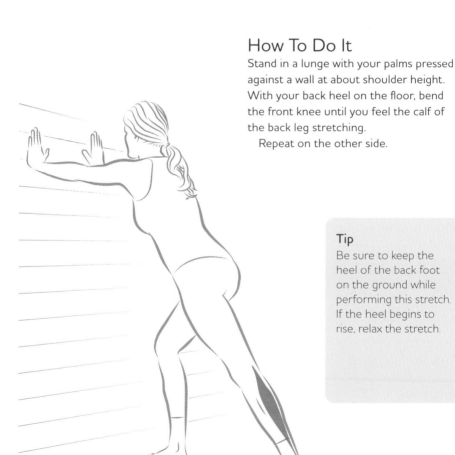

How To Do It

Stand in a lunge with your palms pressed against a wall at about shoulder height. With your back heel on the floor, bend the front knee until you feel the calf of the back leg stretching.

Repeat on the other side.

Tip

Be sure to keep the heel of the back foot on the ground while performing this stretch. If the heel begins to rise, relax the stretch.

2

Calf Stretch Wall

Take your time to find the correct angle for how your foot should be placed against the wall. When you begin to feel the calf stretching, you will know you are in the right place.

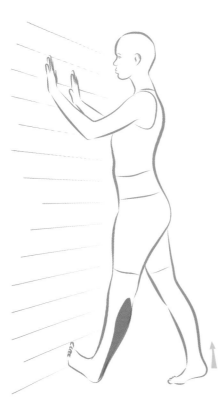

How To Do It

Stand with your palms pressed against a wall at roughly shoulder height. Place the ball of one foot against the wall. Lift the heel of the back foot off the floor until you feel the calf of the front leg stretching.

Repeat on the other side.

Further Considerations

For some people, it may be enough to simply place the front foot against the wall without lifting the back heel. Only stretch to a point that feels comfortable.

3

Tibialis Anterior Stretch

This stretch is particularly useful for any pain or tenderness felt along the front of the shin and foot.

How To Do It

Standing with your hands resting on the back of a chair, place the top of one foot on the floor. Lean forward on this foot until you feel the stretch in the shin area.

Repeat on the other side.

Further Considerations

For many people, placing the top of the foot onto the floor can be stretch enough. Start slowly and don't overdo it.

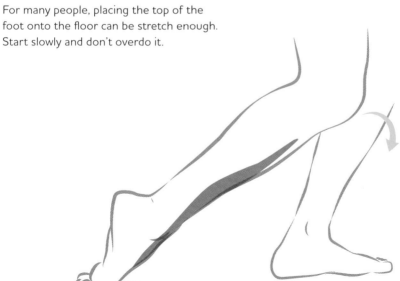

4

Peroneal Stretch

Stretches of the foot can be incredibly relieving, but also tricky to get right. Don't be surprised if you need to adjust the position of your foot to find the sweet spot.

How To Do It

Stand with one foot rolled onto its outside edge.

Repeat on the other side.

Further Considerations

Due to widespread foot pronation, ankle strains/sprains are relatively common injuries. Only roll onto the side of the foot as far as you feel the stretch engage.

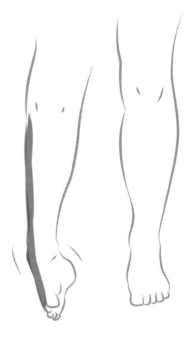

Tip

Use a countertop or chair to ensure that you are not putting any weight on the rolled foot. This is not a weight-bearing stretch.

5

Sitting on Heels

While this sitting posture is found in many Eastern cultures, for Westerners it can be quite uncomfortable. There is no shame in using a bolster to ease any discomfort!

How To Do It

Sit on your heels with the tops of your feet pressing into the floor.

Tip
Place a bolster either between your heels and butt, or spread your feet wide enough to place a bolster between them. This will help relieve any strain on the front side of your lower legs.

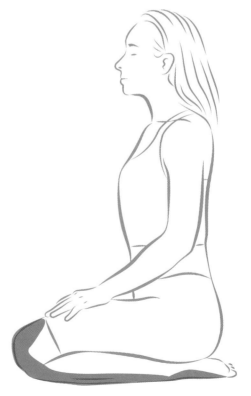

STRETCHES FOR THE
ANKLES, FEET, AND TOES

1

Achilles Stretch

While everyone can benefit from this stretch, anyone who wears high heels will find it particularly rewarding. If that's you, be especially gentle at first. Your Achilles tendon is most likely already in contraction!

How To Do It

Place one foot on a step with your heel hanging off the edge. Allow the heel to drop down below the edge of the step until you feel the Achilles tendon lengthening.

Repeat with the other foot.

Further Considerations

This can be a very intense stretch. Always brace yourself by holding onto a railing to keep from overstretching the calf muscle or possibly injuring the Achilles tendon.

Tip
Use the leg of the stable foot to bring yourself back up to a neutral position.

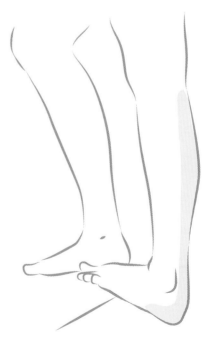

2

Inversion of the Foot

Properly mobile ankles are incredibly important when it comes to dispersing the impact on the feet from walking and running.

How To Do It

Sit with one ankle resting on the opposite knee. With both hands, take hold of the resting foot, placing your thumb on the sole of the foot. Gently turn the foot so the sole is facing up.

Repeat with the other foot.

Further Considerations

Due to widespread foot pronation, many people find it easy to roll their foot so the sole is facing up. Only turn the foot as far as you feel the stretch engage.

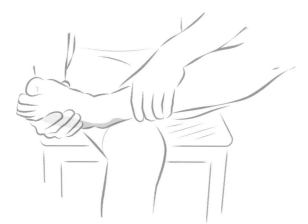

Tip
When turning the foot you may need to slightly twist the direction to feel the stretch. You can make subtle adjustments once the stretch is engaged to feel more of the benefits.

3

Eversion of the Foot

If you find this stretch hard to access, you're not alone. Most people's feet evert only slightly. That's normal. Do not overdo it.

How To Do It

Sit with one ankle resting on the opposite knee. Take hold of the resting foot with your fingers wrapped around the sole. Gently turn the foot so the ball begins to face the floor.

Repeat with the other foot.

Tip

Begin with a gentle twisting of the foot, and slowly increase the force just to the point of feeling the stretching sensation.

Further Considerations

There is considerably more flexibility when inverting the foot (see opposite) versus everting it. Do not be surprised if the foot turns only a little, even when applying slightly more force.

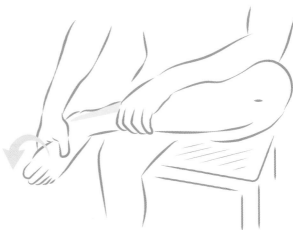

4

Plantar Fascia Stretch

Plantar fasciitis is one of the most common pathologies that affects people's feet. This stretch is crucial in any sort of rehab for the condition.

How To Do It

While standing, come onto the ball of one foot.

Repeat with the other foot.

Alternative

If you are flexible enough, you can achieve a deeper plantar fascia stretch by sitting on your heels with the balls of both feet on the floor. Keep your hands planted in front of you to moderate how deep you go.

Tip

The knee of the stretched foot will naturally bend. Lean slightly forward toward the bent knee to increase the stretch.

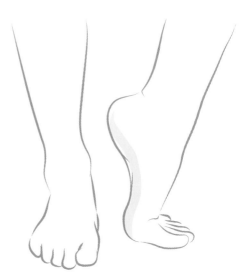

5

Toe Flexion

Stretching the tops of the toes is one of the easiest and most rewarding stretches you can do for those industrious little piggies (or "digits," but piggies is funnier and harks back to the famous nursery rhyme).

How To Do It

While sitting in a chair, bring one heel up and place the tops of the toes on the floor. Press the tops of the toes into the floor until you feel the stretch engage.

Repeat with the other foot.

Alternative

You can also stretch the toes individually with your hands (see page 95).

Tips

Coming slightly onto the top of the foot will increase the stretch.

It is preferable to do this stretch barefoot or in socks.

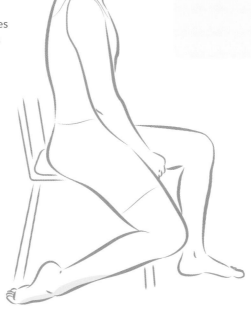

6

Toe Extension

Stretching the roots of the toes just above the ball of the foot can have you experiencing relief far beyond the foot.

How To Do It

While sitting in a chair, bring one heel up until the ball of the foot is resting on the floor. Press the bottoms of the toes into the floor until you feel the stretch engage.
  Repeat with the other foot.

Alternative

You can also stretch the toes individually with your hands (see opposite).

Tip
It is preferable to do this stretch barefoot or in socks.

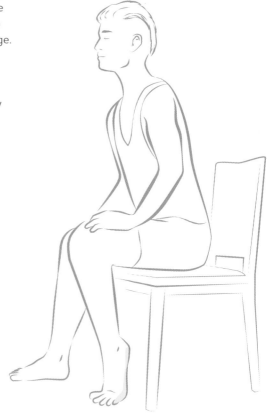

7

Toe Spreading

Modern conventional shoes tend to strangle the toes. Walking barefoot, along with stretching the toes, can provide incredible relief for tight, overworked feet.

How To Do It

Take hold of two toes, one in each hand, and gently pull them apart from one another.

Repeat with the other toes and on the other foot.

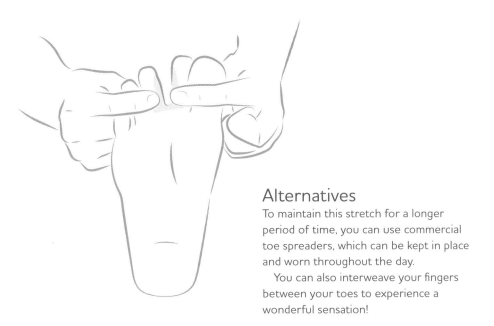

Alternatives

To maintain this stretch for a longer period of time, you can use commercial toe spreaders, which can be kept in place and worn throughout the day.

You can also interweave your fingers between your toes to experience a wonderful sensation!

Spreading Top and Bottom of Foot

Because modern shoes tend to restrict the organic and dynamic movement of the feet, stretching them often is an important practice.

How To Do It

Take hold of one of your feet with both hands, wrapping the fingers around the bottom of the foot. Slowly stretch the top and bottom of the foot by bending the foot down the middle.

Repeat with the other foot.

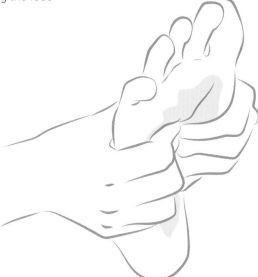

Tip

Allowing the hands to slowly drag across the skin will add an extra layer of stretch to the overall technique.

9

Tennis Ball Stretch

While technically not a stretch, using a tennis ball to lengthen and massage the bottom of your feet can be very satisfying and therapeutic.

How To Do It

While either sitting or standing, place a tennis ball under your foot. Apply just enough pressure on the ball to feel the tissue of your foot soften.

Repeat with the other foot.

Further Considerations

Slowly roll your foot over the ball, taking time to pause when you feel an area of particular tenderness.

Tip

If you find an area that is particularly tender, and you feel as if a bit more pressure might be beneficial, engage the muscles in that area. This will stiffen the muscles, but can have the effect of making the pressure more acute.

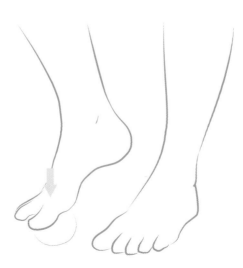

CHAPTER 3
WHICH STRETCHES TO USE

Use this chapter to target your needs with the relevant stretches. The first section looks at a selection of occupational and sports-related activities and considers the ways they affect our bodies. The second section looks at specific areas of the body where pain may be felt. Find out how the activity or injury relates to the body, then use the selection of stretches to help improve your performance, or for rehabilitation.

STRETCHES FOR
ACTIVITIES

Sitting All Day

We are often warned about the dangers of sedentary lifestyles. Weight gain (particularly around the waistline), high blood sugar, high blood pressure, and an increased risk of heart disease and even cancer have all been linked to a lifestyle revolving around long periods of sitting. Low back pain is also a very common and immediate response to sitting all day.

When standing, there is roughly 2–3 feet (0.5–1m) of legs (depending on your age and height) buffering the low back from the force of gravity above and the resistance of the Earth below. Our bodies have been engineered over hundreds of thousands of years to gracefully navigate this pressure.

When we sit, we take our evolutionary successes and replace them with a manufactured object— such as a chair. In short stints, any seat can be a pleasant respite for the legs. However, when we sit for hours each day (you may be sitting upward of 10 to 13 hours a day!), no amount of manufactured ergonomic mastery can make up for what our bodies can do through stretching and movement.

STRETCHES

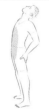

Ab Stretch
Page 61

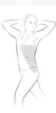

Ab Twist
Page 62

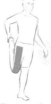

Runner's Stretch
Page 76

Supta Vajrasana
Page 77

Seated Forward Fold
Page 78

Standing All Day

While not as detrimental to our health as sitting all day, standing for extended periods of time comes with its own set of concerns, typically in the form of aches and pains throughout the body, but especially in the low back, feet, and joints.

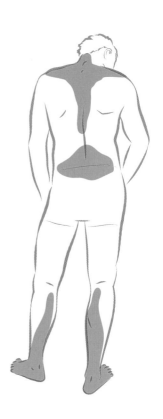

Those with professions that require standing or walking slowly all day—security guards, foot patrol, etc.—can feel extreme tightness in the lumbar region, throbbing pain in the feet, and restless aches in the shoulders.

Along with proper (lightweight if possible) footwear, and supportive straps for heavy belts, stretching before, after, and during your shift should become a regular habit.

STRETCHES

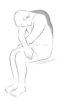

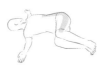

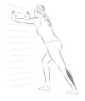

Trapezius Stretch
Page 46

Double Knees Across Twist
Page 71

Ankle to Knee
Page 73

Calf Stretch Lunge
Page 83

Spreading Top and Bottom of Foot
Page 96

Walking

While research continues to prove the many benefits of walking every day, as with any body-centered activity, mild discomfort can also be present. Even the most efficient walker is still subject to potential aches in the joints, feet, and legs, and knowing how to condition, and especially stretch, your hips, knees, calves, and feet can have incredibly relieving effects on the body.

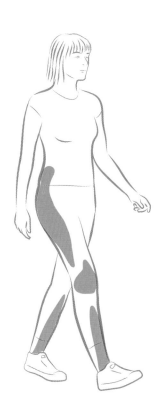

No matter what your level of proficiency in this seemingly innocent activity, when you walk your knees feel the effects of one-and-a-half times your body weight with every step. This means that a 150-pound (68-kg) person experiences 225 pounds (102kg) of pressure on each knee with every step. And that's on level ground! This load increases with any sort of incline.

STRETCHES

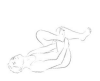

Ankle to Knee
Page 73

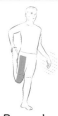

Runner's Stretch
Page 76

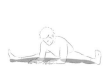

Seated Wide Leg
Page 80

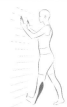

Calf Stretch Wall
Page 84

Plantar Fascia Stretch
Page 92

Driving Long Distances

Anyone who drives long distances or regularly spends time in traffic knows how grueling sitting in a car can be. While passengers may experience general aches and pains from the same drive, the driver's body is prone to specific areas of discomfort.

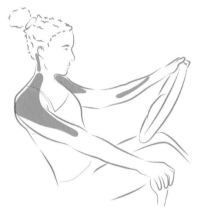

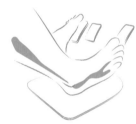

Even though you are using the wheel as a shelf, of sorts, for your arms to rest on, the arms still need to be elevated in order to make quick turns and be on the alert. This means that the shoulders can become quite tired.

Keeping one or both feet in dorsiflexion when using the pedals puts a great deal of strain on both the calves and feet. Imagine keeping your feet in this position while not driving and you'll realize right away how uncomfortable this is.

STRETCHES

Head Back Stretch
Page 36

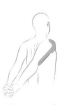

Pectoralis Stretch
Page 41

Ankle to Knee
Page 73

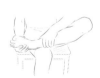

Inversion of the Foot
Page 90

Calf Stretch Wall
Page 84

Lifting, Carrying, Carting

When picking things up you have no doubt heard the admonition to "lift with your legs." While lifting with the legs is exactly what you should be doing, doing this all day will inevitably lead to aches and pains, and potential chronic conditions. People who are required to lift, cart, and carry deal with specific pain patterns unique to their labor. Neck pain, low back pain, and tired and weak arms and legs are all notable culprits.

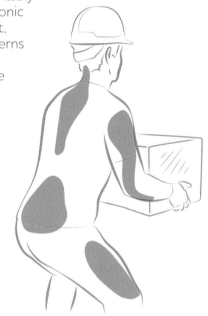

Maintaining perfect alignment and ergonomics throughout the day for any activity is next to impossible. Inevitably, your attention wanders or you get tired, and slowly your good intentions start to fall by the wayside. At these times you are prone to injury and the aches and pains associated with repetitive stressors.

STRETCHES

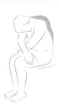

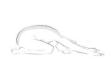

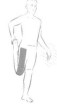

Chin to Sternum
Page 35

Trapezius Stretch
Page 46

Child's Pose
Page 68

Knee Across Twist
Page 74

Runner's Stretch
Page 76

Texting

Constant smartphone use, and especially texting, is one of the leading causes of what has been dubbed texting thumb, which is experienced as pain extending around the entire base of the thumb. Add to this the pain associated with the commonly held chin-to-chest positioning of the head while texting, and you can easily see how potentially harmful this seemingly innocent activity can be.

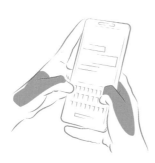

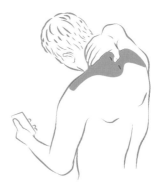

The repetitive up-down motion of the thumbs causes strain and pain around the joint, as well as in the muscles and tendons.

Constantly looking down at your phone dramatically increases your chances of feeling aches in the back, neck, and shoulder muscles. Over time, these aches can turn into chronic conditions, which may require a great deal of massage and physical therapy in the future.

STRETCHES

Eye Stretches
Page 25

Looking into the Distance
Page 26

Traction Below the Collarbone
Page 34

Palms Out Stretch
Page 55

De Quervain's Stretch
Page 59

Staring at Screens

Screens are ubiquitous. They are our phones, our computers, our alarm clocks, our televisions, our instructors, even our workout buddies (think yoga at home!). New patterns of discomfort and pathologies are being discovered all the time related to our level of screen usage.

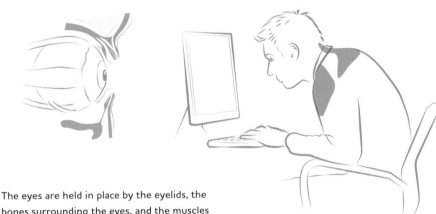

The eyes are held in place by the eyelids, the bones surrounding the eyes, and the muscles attached to the eyes and bones. These muscles also help keep the eyes in one position and the eyelids open, both of which we do for extended periods of time while looking at screens.

Sitting at a desk all day promotes various kinds of slouched postures, which inevitably leads to aches along the back, neck, and shoulders.

STRETCHES

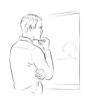

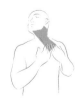

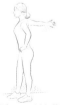

Eye Stretches
Page 25

Looking into the Distance
Page 26

Traction Below the Collarbone
Page 34

Biceps Wall Stretch
Page 50

Tented Fingers
Page 56

Running

Is running just walking fast? Shouldn't we simply stretch the same muscles for running as we would for walking? The answer to both of these questions is "yes" and "no." Yes, because on a very basic level you use similar muscle groups when you walk and run, and, yes, a gentle walk sped up can become a jog, which in turn can become a run. There are, however, a number of very important differences which make running and jogging specific exercises that are different from walking.

One of the main differences between walking and running is that there is an "airborne phase" in running, when both feet are actually not touching the ground. This occurs between the back foot pushing off the ground and the front foot landing. Imagine all the muscles having to engage and resist the added force that comes with replanting the feet on the ground after liftoff: four to eight times your body weight translates through your foot and into your knees when running.

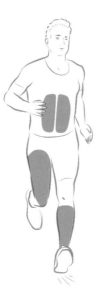

The muscles in the abdomen and low back work to keep you erect, and the muscles in the shoulders jostle while hugging your arms close to your body, so it is important to comprehensively stretch the body after a run.

STRETCHES

Outside Hip Stretch
Page 75

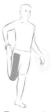

Runner's Stretch
Page 76

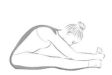

Seated Forward Fold
Page 78

Calf Stretch Lunge
Page 83

Tibialis Anterior Stretch
Page 85

Cycling

While on the surface it's easy to assume that cycling is primarily a leg activity (and in many ways it is), a lot more goes into making our bikes do what we want them to. Consequently, when stretching as it relates to cycling, you will also focus on other areas of the body.

In order to keep yourself balanced and moving forward when riding you continuously flex and extend the upper legs, which builds strength in the legs and hips, but also creates tightness.

Anyone who's ever gone on an extended bike ride can attest not only to soreness in the legs, but also to tenderness in the shoulders and neck, and palms. Propping yourself up on the handlebars will inevitably lead to some general aches and pains in these areas.

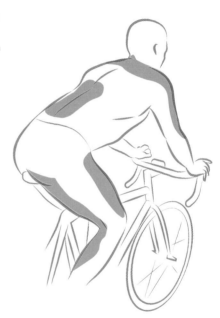

STRETCHES

Chin to Sternum
Page 35

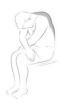

Trapezius Stretch
Page 46

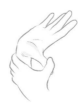

Thumb Stretch Down
Page 57

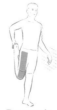

Runner's Stretch
Page 76

Calf Stretch Lunge
Page 83

Swimming

While not a load-bearing exercise, swimming is a wonderful conditioning activity that engages the shoulders, arms, and legs in a very dynamic way. Swimming does not put pressure on the bones, and is thus not useful for developing bone density and strength. However, this activity engages many large muscle groups that will need stretching.

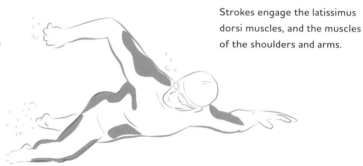

Swimming involves constant repetitive motions of both the legs and the arms.

Strokes engage the latissimus dorsi muscles, and the muscles of the shoulders and arms.

Kicking propels you from behind using your strong upper leg muscles, as well as the muscles of the lower legs and feet (think of how many micro and not-so-micro movements the feet make when kicking through the water).

The muscles of the back and abdomen engage to keep you on a relatively flat plane as you glide through the water.

STRETCHES

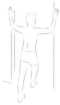

Doorway Pectoralis Stretch
Page 42

Chest Stretch
Page 44

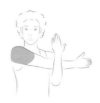

Deltoid Stretch
Page 45

Forward Fold
Page 67

Supta Vajrasana
Page 77

Surfing

You might typically imagine a surfer gracefully gliding and turning down the face of a rippleless wave. In turn, you might think that the aches and pains associated with surfing would concentrate around the legs. While issues with the knees and quadricep muscles are certainly common, surfers are often more concerned with their shoulders and low back.

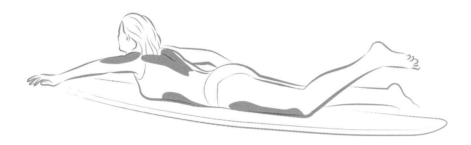

The surfing part of surfing is, in a way, a small portion of what goes into the art form. Paddling to catch waves, as well as "popping up" to stand on the board, are often what causes the most nagging of issues.

STRETCHES

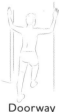

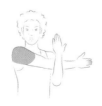

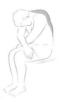

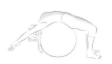

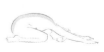

Doorway Pectoralis Stretch
Page 42

Deltoid Stretch
Page 45

Trapezius Stretch
Page 46

Stability Ball Stretch
Page 63

Child's Pose
Page 68

Skiing

Although the most amount of pain related to skiing activities might come from a fall, anyone new to the sport can attest that a number of aches come with simply performing the activity.

So much of skiing has to do with the position of the legs. Skiers use their legs to turn and maneuver, to decrease in speed, and come to full stops.

Ski boots, although intended to be protective of the feet and ankles, often cause aches because of how secure and immobilized the feet and ankles are while wearing them.

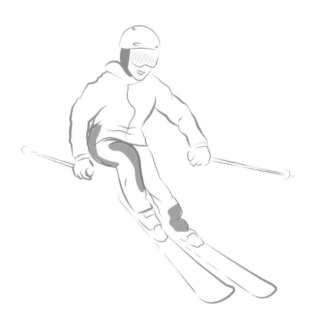

STRETCHES

Knees to Chest
Page 69

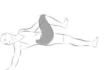

Knee Across Twist
Page 74

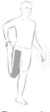

Runner's Stretch
Page 76

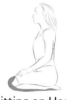

Sitting on Heels
Page 87

Spreading Top and Bottom of Foot
Page 96

Skateboarding and Snowboarding

While skateboarding and snowboarding are considerably different sports—not the least of which has to do with the fact that in snowboarding your feet are locked in place—both share some commonalities in the ways in which people hold their bodies.

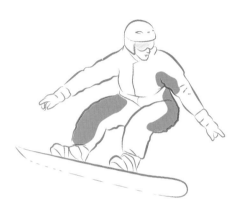

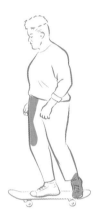

Casual skateboarding and snowboarding will primarily involve a sustained posture in which the knees are bent with the feet placed slightly at an angle, which over time can cause pain and discomfort in the knees and hips.

Skateboarding has the added effect of propulsion by swinging one leg and kicking off the ground. This repetitive motion commonly causes pain and discomfort in the Achilles tendon and the plantar fascia, as well as in the upper (dorsal) side of the foot, especially where the foot meets the leg.

STRETCHES

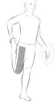

Runner's Stretch
Page 76

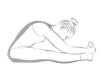

Seated Forward Fold
Page 78

Adductors Stretch
Page 79

Calf Stretch Lunge
Page 83

Plantar Fascia Stretch
Page 92

Hiking

Urban and suburban lifestyles have mostly done away with any inconsistencies in our bipedal travels. Surfaces are mainly flat, organized, and free of obstructions. Hiking in nature gives the body, and especially the feet, an opportunity to actually work as they navigate uneven surfaces and protrusions from the earth.

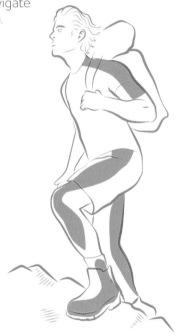

Walking over roots and rocks, and up and down inclines and declines; having to propel yourself over fallen trees with your legs; and dropping down from higher points to lower points will involve your entire body. This is part of what makes hiking so exhilarating. However, the brunt of much of what's involved in hiking falls on the legs, ankles, and feet.

Descending down a mountainside will call on the hip flexors and leg extensors, quads and glutes, and flexors and extensors of the feet. Inclines will do much the same, but you'll be using your arms and the muscles on the front side of your legs a lot more!

STRETCHES

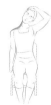

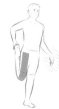

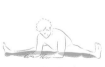

Lateral Neck Stretch	Deltoid Stretch	Knees to Chest	Runner's Stretch	Seated Wide Leg
Page 37	*Page 45*	*Page 69*	*Page 76*	*Page 80*

Rock Climbing

Rock climbing is such a comprehensive sport that in some ways, when thinking about what to stretch for it, it's actually easier to think about what NOT to stretch.

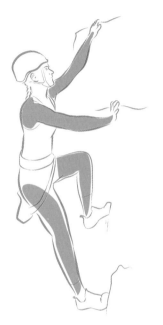

Muscles are engaged almost everywhere imaginable when climbing, and especially around the upper and lower legs, the shoulders, and the entire length of the arms.

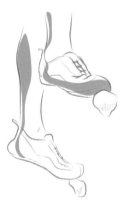

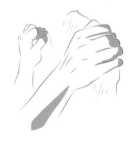

In addition to the myriad muscle groups working while climbing, the unsung heroes of the sport are the fingers and toes, which all need to be both flexible and strong.

STRETCHES

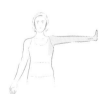

Full Arm Wall Stretch
Page 51

Palms Out Stretch
Page 55

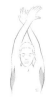

Latissimus Dorsi Stretch
Page 70

Calf Stretch Lunge
Page 83

Spreading Top and Bottom of Foot
Page 96

STRETCHES FOR

ACHES AND PAINS

Head and Neck Pain

Head and neck pain can present itself anywhere, from the top of the head, down around the entire neck, and even into the muscle tissue between the shoulders and base of the neck. Like most pain patterns, discomfort can radiate, or refer, to different areas within the region.

For many people, head and neck pain often arises after sleeping in an uncomfortable position for too long, or from tension headaches, both of which can initiate pain in other immediate areas of the body.

STRETCHES

Traction Below the Collarbone
Page 34

Chin to Sternum
Page 35

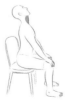

Head Back Stretch
Page 36

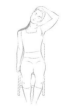

Lateral Neck Stretch
Page 37

Toward the Armpit
Page 38

Shoulder Pain

Shoulder pain may be described as any pain or discomfort extending from the base of the neck, across the front side of the shoulder, around the deltoid muscle, and across the shoulder blade. Some of the most common causes of shoulder pain are due to sleeping in an uncomfortable position for too long, repetitive stress activities such as sports and labor-intensive jobs, and minor tears caused by all of the above.

Other conditions that may require more attention from a physician are dislocations of the shoulder; overstretched, irritated, or torn muscles, tendons, or ligaments; strains and sprains; bursitis; arthritis; rotary cuff injuries; and frozen shoulder associated with any of the above.

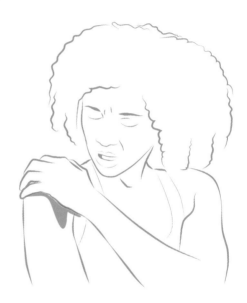

STRETCHES

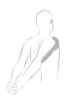

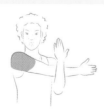

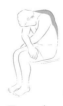

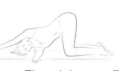

Pectoralis Stretch
Page 41

Deltoid Stretch
Page 45

Trapezius Stretch
Page 46

Thread the Needle
Page 47

Triceps Stretch
Page 49

Elbow Pain

Elbow pain typically manifests on the elbow itself, or near, or directly on, the bony protuberances found on either side of the elbow. Elbow pain is often attributed to either trauma (i.e. falling onto your elbow) or repetitive stress from laborious activities and sports involving swinging or rotating the arms.

One of the sneakier causes of elbow pain involves resting your elbows on a desk or table for long periods of time. While this may seem inconsequential or even obvious, many people unknowingly cause themselves unnecessary pain through repeating this activity.

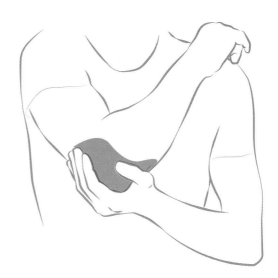

STRETCHES

Triceps Stretch
Page 49

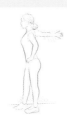

Biceps Wall Stretch
Page 50

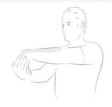

Forearm Extensor Stretch
Page 52

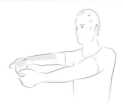

Forearm Flexor Stretch
Page 53

Hand and Wrist Pain

For many people, pain in the hand and wrist immediately equates to carpel tunnel syndrome. While in some cases that may be true, hand and wrist pain can have at its root many causes.

Performing muscle tests under the guidance of a bodywork practitioner can help to identify the specific pathology causing pain in the hand and wrist—often general tendon pain, sometimes called tendonosis, is the issue.

Due to overuse (especially from texting and typing), a series of very small tears (microtears) in the tissue in or around the tendons of the forearm and wrist can, over time, cause irritation and pain.

In addition to pain and tenderness, common symptoms of tendon injury include decreased strength and movement in the affected area.

Because many of the strongest muscles of the hand and wrist begin in the forearm, stretching the muscles of the forearm is an integral part of any relief to the hand and wrist

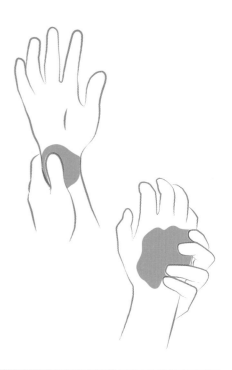

STRETCHES

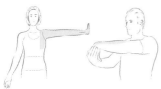

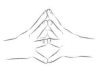

Full Arm Wall Stretch
Page 51

Forearm Extensor Stretch
Page 52

Forearm Flexor Stretch
Page 53

Wrist Stretch
Page 54

Tented Fingers
Page 56

Low Back Pain

Low back pain can be described as any pain or discomfort in the lumbar region. People may experience pain or discomfort when sitting, standing, bending over, and stretching, translated often as either shooting/stabbing pain or a general dull achiness.

Low back pain can have a myriad of physiological causes, including slipped or herniated discs and overused muscles.

The kind of back pain that follows heavy lifting or exercising too hard is often caused by muscle strain.

Sometimes back pain is related to a disc that bulges or ruptures, and if this presses on the sciatic nerve, pain may run from the buttock down one or both legs. This pressure on the root of the sciatic nerve is called sciatica.

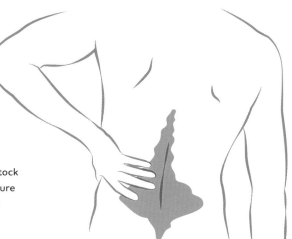

STRETCHES

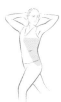

Ab Twist
Page 62

Side Stretch with Twist
Page 66

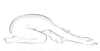

Child's Pose
Page 68

Knees to Chest
Page 69

Ankle to Knee
Page 73

Hip and Groin Pain

While pain in the hip and groin are very distinct from one another, in many cases we end up stretching and massaging both when there's discomfort in either of the two areas. Not only is this because of the close proximity of the two, but also because of the interconnected relationship between these two regions of the body.

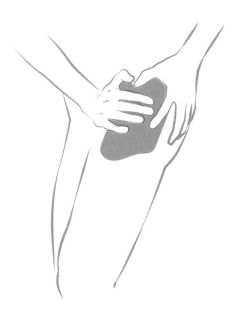

In younger people hip and groin injuries are often the result of playing sports that involve running or sprinting, stopping, and shifts in weight from side to side. Soccer and football are common activities that inflict frequent pain in the hip and groin.

In older communities, pain in the hip is often the result of overuse and arthritis, both of which have the effect of breaking down the protective cartilage that surrounds the head of the femur. This degeneration leads to rubbing of the bone in the hip socket, which usually causes considerable to extreme discomfort.

STRETCHES

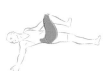

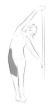

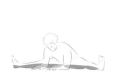

Ankle to Knee
Page 73

Knee Across Twist
Page 74

Outside Hip Stretch
Page 75

Seated Wide Leg
Page 80

Adductors Side Lunge
Page 81

Knee Pain

Knee pain can be described as any pain present around the knee, including above and below the patella, on either side of the knee, as well as in the soft tissue behind the knee. In order to plan an effective treatment or stretching session, it's incredibly important to have a clear sense of where the pain is located, as well as what muscles or regions of the leg or hip might be causing the discomfort.

To list and evaluate the potential causes of knee pain would take an entire book, and so is a bit beyond the scope of these pages. However, there are a few common sources we can look at.

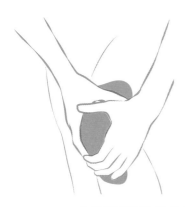

Patellar tracking syndrome is a common pathology that usually involves a tight iliotibial band tracking the patella toward the outside of the leg. This misalignment can lead to a deterioration of cartilaginous tissue under the patella, as well as clicking sounds and general discomfort.

Meniscus tears are common in athletes or anyone who engages in activities that involve running, short stops, and quick turns. During these activities pressure is added to the half-moon-shaped, spongy meniscus pads that buffer the strong femur and tibia bones of the upper and lower legs, which will sometimes lead to tears in the meniscus.

STRETCHES

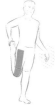

Runner's Stretch
Page 76

Supta Vajrasana
Page 77

Adductors Side Lunge
Page 81

Calf Stretch Lunge
Page 83

Tibialis Anterior Stretch
Page 85

Ankle and Foot Pain

Whether standing, leaning, walking, or running, our feet are our primary contact points with the ground. Not only do they help to keep us balanced, but our feet also take in information from whatever we are standing on and translate the force into the rest of the body, starting with the complex joints of the ankles.

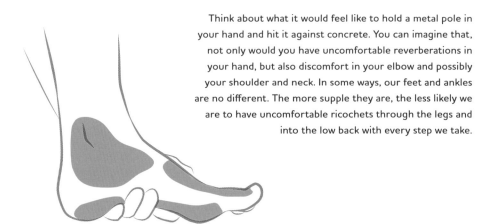

Think about what it would feel like to hold a metal pole in your hand and hit it against concrete. You can imagine that, not only would you have uncomfortable reverberations in your hand, but also discomfort in your elbow and possibly your shoulder and neck. In some ways, our feet and ankles are no different. The more supple they are, the less likely we are to have uncomfortable ricochets through the legs and into the low back with every step we take.

Tight feet and ankles are much more prone to injury, as well as increased discomfort in the knees and low back.

STRETCHES

**Calf Stretch
Lunge**
Page 83

**Tibialis Anterior
Stretch**
Page 85

**Peroneal
Stretch**
Page 86

**Plantar Fascia
Stretch**
Page 92

**Spreading Top
and Bottom
of Foot**
Page 96

Stress

There are two types of stress: eustress and distress. Feeling overworked, drained, worn out, and anxious are all typically interpreted as forms of distress. Eustress, on the other hand, is positive stress. It's the stress that, although at times difficult to navigate, ultimately leads us to a more beneficial place in our lives. Buying a home, having a child, and exercise are all forms of eustress.

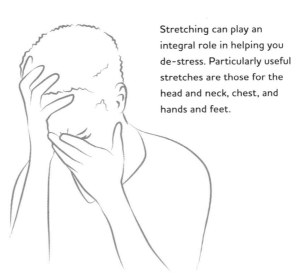

Stretching is a form of eustress where we exert physical energy in order to increase our wellbeing. When it comes to our bodies, we use intentional (eu)stressors to combat the disstressors.

Anything from anxiety disorders, mental illness, and digestion and cardiovascular issues, as well as a decrease in the rate of healing, can be attributed to prolonged bouts of distress.

Stretching can play an integral role in helping you de-stress. Particularly useful stretches are those for the head and neck, chest, and hands and feet.

STRETCHES

Around the Eyes
Page 28

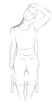

Lateral Neck Stretch
Page 37

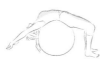

Stability Ball Stretch
Page 63

Double Knees Across Twist
Page 71

Spreading Top and Bottom of Foot
Page 96

Index